Cambridge Discover

▶ **INTERACTIVE**

Series editor: Bob

C000254094

DO NOT DISTURB
THE IMPORTANCE
OF SLEEP

A1⁺

Genevieve Kocienda

CAMBRIDGE
UNIVERSITY PRESS

Discovery
EDUCATION

CAMBRIDGE UNIVERSITY PRESS
Cambridge, New York, Melbourne, Madrid, Cape Town,
Singapore, São Paulo, Delhi, Mexico City

Cambridge University Press
32 Avenue of the Americas, New York, NY 10013-2473, USA

www.cambridge.org
Information on this title: www.cambridge.org/9781107646827

© Cambridge University Press 2014

First published 2014

Printed in Hong Kong, China, by Golden Cup Printing Company Limited

A catalog record for this publication is available from the British Library.

Library of Congress Cataloging-in-Publication Data

Kocienda, G.
  Do not disturb : the importance of sleep / Genevieve Kocienda.
      pages cm. -- (Cambridge discovery interactive readers)
   ISBN 978-1-107-64682-7 (pbk. : alk. paper)
   1. Sleep--Juvenile literature. 2. English language--Textbooks for foreign speakers. 3. Readers
(Elementary) I. Title.

QP425.K58 2013
612.8'21--dc23

2013024754

ISBN 978-1-107-64682-7

Additional resources for this publication at www.cambridge.org

Layout services, art direction, book design, and photo research: Q2ABillSMITH GROUP
Editorial services: Hyphen S.A.
Audio production: CityVox, New York
Video production: Q2ABillSMITH GROUP

Contents

Before You Read: Get Ready!

Sleep is important for our health. Some people need a lot of sleep; others need very little. But we all need sleep to feel good.

Words to Know

Look at the pictures. Then complete the sentences below with the correct words.

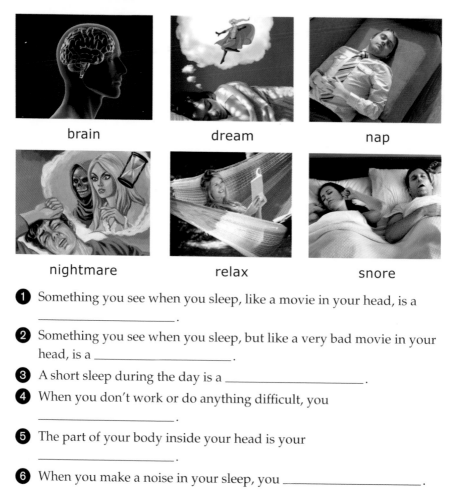

brain   dream   nap

nightmare   relax   snore

1 Something you see when you sleep, like a movie in your head, is a

_____.

2 Something you see when you sleep, but like a very bad movie in your head, is a _____.

3 A short sleep during the day is a _____.

4 When you don't work or do anything difficult, you

_____.

5 The part of your body inside your head is your

_____.

6 When you make a noise in your sleep, you _____.

Words to Know

**Read the paragraph. Then complete the sentences below
with the correct highlighted words.**

Last night, I did not sleep well. I closed my eyes, but I did not
fall asleep. I was awake until 2:00 a.m. My mind was very busy. So now,
I don't feel rested. I feel very tired and sleepy, but I have to go to school!

1 When you're not sleeping, you are _____.

2 When you are _____, you don't feel tired.

3 Your _____ is all the things that you feel, know,
remember, and think about.

4 When you're tired and need to sleep, you are _____.

5 When you _____, you begin to sleep.

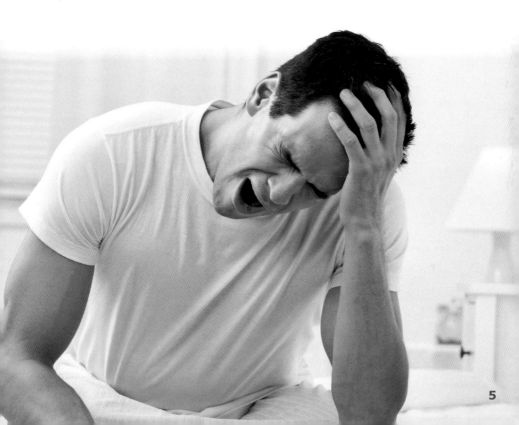

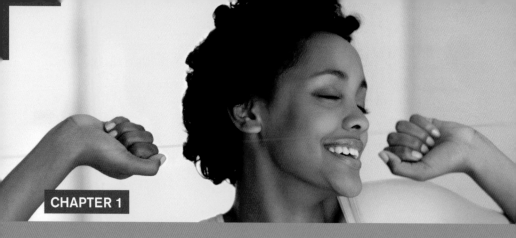

CHAPTER 1

Get Your Sleep

WE SPEND ABOUT ONE THIRD OF OUR TIME SLEEPING – THAT'S ABOUT 122 DAYS A YEAR!

Why do we need to sleep? And why do we need to sleep so much? Scientists think that maybe we need sleep to help our bodies repair[1] themselves.

Think about how you feel when you're tired. It is difficult to think, work, talk, or walk. Now, think about how your body feels when you're well rested. You feel better.

In the daytime, your body uses a lot of energy.[2] When you sleep, you get more energy. Your body needs sleep like a car needs gas.

[1] **repair:** make something work again when it's broken
[2] **energy:** You have energy when you are doing a lot of things and feel good.

So, how much sleep do we need? Most adults need 7 to 9 hours of sleep a night. But some people need a lot more. New babies need 16 hours a day. Older babies need 12 to 14 hours. Teenagers need about 9 hours. Pregnant[3] women in the first three months of pregnancy need more sleep than other women.

Some people don't need much sleep. For example, the artist Pablo Picasso usually slept only 2 to 4 hours a night. Leonardo da Vinci slept only 1 to 2 hours a night! But he did take short 15-minute naps every 4 hours.

One man wanted to see how long it was possible to stay awake. Toimi Soini, from Finland, stayed awake for 276 hours!

[3] **pregnant:** A pregnant woman is going to have a baby.

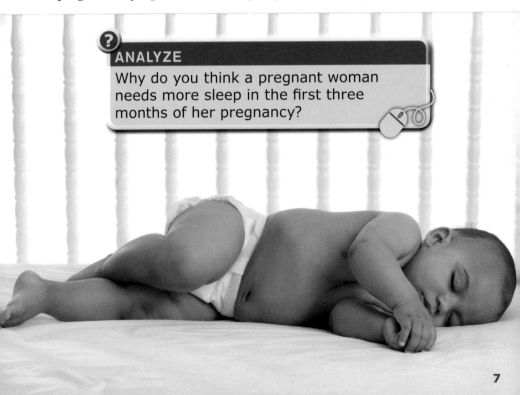

? ANALYZE

Why do you think a pregnant woman needs more sleep in the first three months of her pregnancy?

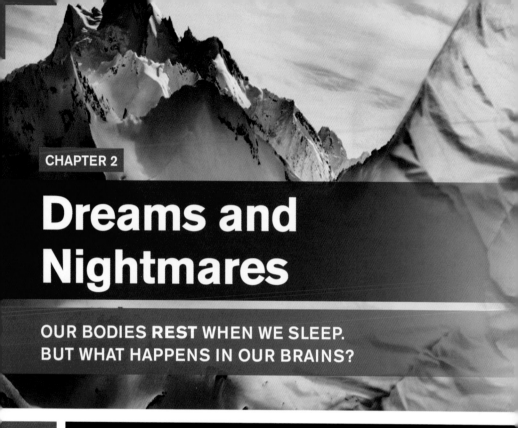

CHAPTER 2

Dreams and Nightmares

OUR BODIES **REST** WHEN WE SLEEP.
BUT WHAT HAPPENS IN OUR BRAINS?

There are two different kinds of sleep – **REM sleep** and non-REM sleep. In non-REM sleep, our bodies get the energy we need to live. In this kind of sleep, we don't usually **dream**. It is easy to wake up from non-REM sleep. But when you wake up from non-REM sleep, you feel sleepy; you don't feel awake and rested.

REM sleep is different. REM is short for "rapid eye movement." In REM sleep your eyes **move** a lot, and they move very fast. This shows that your brain is working hard. It is in REM sleep that we have **dreams** – or nightmares.

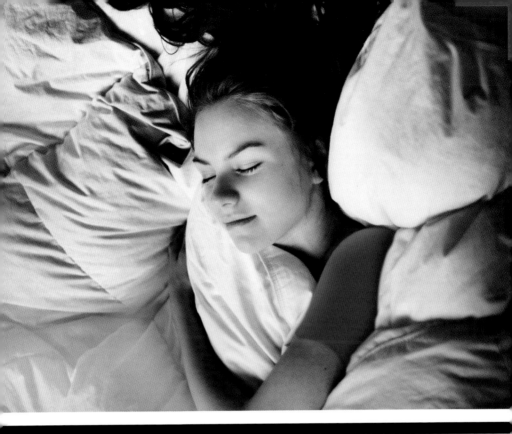

Everybody dreams. Do you remember your dreams? Maybe you don't, but you dream every night. Your first dreams of the night are very short, but then they get longer and longer. Your first dream is about 10 minutes long. Your last dream, before you wake up in the morning, is about 45 minutes long.

Your dreams help you remember and learn things. When you study, one part of your brain works. When you dream, the same part of your brain works. So, when you want to learn something new, don't study too long. Take a nap. It can help you learn!

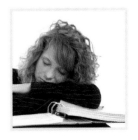

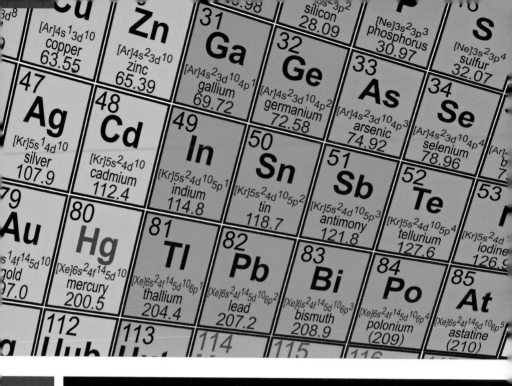

Dreaming can also help you with problems. Dreams can help you see a problem in a new way and find an answer.

For example, one day in February 1869, Russian scientist Dmitri Mendeleev fell asleep. In his dream he saw how to write the Periodic Table! Singer Paul McCartney woke up one morning with the music of the famous Beatles song "Yesterday" in his head.

Painter Salvador Dali often used his dreams for ideas. He always went to sleep with a spoon in his hand. After he fell asleep, the spoon hit the floor and made a noise. He woke up and painted the things from his dreams.

Do dreams mean anything? Some people say that the things in your dream are symbols[4] of what you think and feel in your life. For example:

- a house = your mind. The different rooms in the house are different parts of your mind.

- a road = where your life is going.

- a mountain = a problem in your life.

- hair = your opinion.[5] When you change your hair in your dream, you are changing how you think about something in your life.

How can you remember your dreams? Put a pencil and paper next to your bed. When you wake up, write down your dream. What do you think it means?

[4] **symbol:** something that really means something else
[5] **opinion:** a thought about something or someone

Some people dream of mountains. Maybe they are really dreaming about problems.

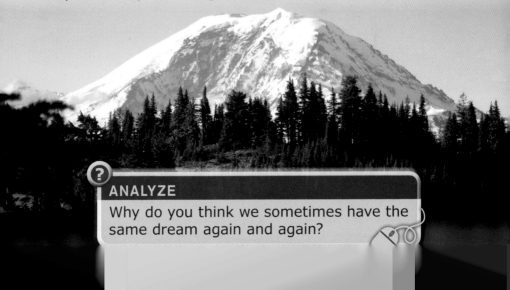

?

ANALYZE
Why do you think we sometimes have the same dream again and again?

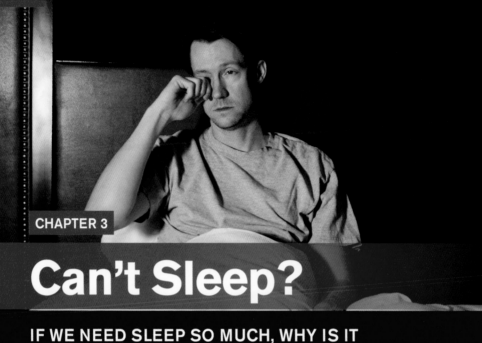

CHAPTER 3

Can't Sleep?

IF WE NEED SLEEP SO MUCH, WHY IS IT SOMETIMES DIFFICULT TO SLEEP?

Sometimes you want to sleep, but you can't. Why? There are many reasons[6] why you don't get enough sleep.

Sometimes you have to stay up late to study or to work. Or maybe someone in your house snores very loudly. Or you live in a noisy place where there are many cars and people outside your window at night. All these things can stop you from getting your **rest**.

When there's no reason, but you still can't sleep, that's insomnia. Most of us have insomnia at some time in our lives. Everything is quiet, you are tired, but you can't sleep.

[6]**reason:** why something happens

It's okay if you can't sleep for a night or two, but it's not good if you don't sleep enough for many nights.

Too little sleep can be bad for your **health**:

- It can make you fat. Often, when people sleep less, they eat more. And they eat bad things, like cake and potato chips.

- It can make you sad and depressed.[7]

- It can give you headaches.

- It can make you sick and make your life shorter!

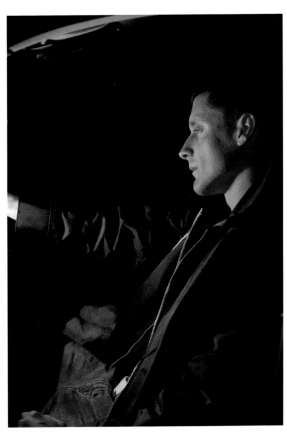

Getting too little sleep can be **dangerous**, too. For example, it is very dangerous to drive a car when you are sleepy.

....

[7] **depressed:** very sad, often for a long time

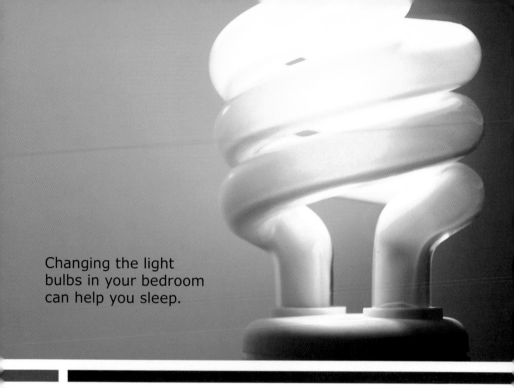

Changing the light bulbs in your bedroom can help you sleep.

So how can you get enough sleep?

First, it is important to go to sleep and wake up at the same time every day.

Don't watch TV or look at your computer before you go to sleep. They stimulate[8] your mind. You can't sleep if you're thinking too much and your mind is not relaxed.

Try changing the light bulbs in your bedroom. Looking at bright[9] lights before bedtime can stop you from sleeping.

Also, a bedroom must not be too warm or too cold. Most people sleep well in a bedroom between 18° and 22° Celsius.

[8] **stimulate:** make excited
[9] **bright:** having a lot of light

Here are more tips[10] for getting a good night's sleep:

❶ Don't eat too much before bedtime. If you're hungry before you go to sleep, have something small to eat.

❷ Before you go to bed, listen to quiet music or read a book to relax your mind.

❸ When you are in bed, close your eyes and **breathe** very slowly. Don't think about problems or worries. Think about a favorite place, like the beach or a beautiful park.

❹ Don't eat or drink anything with caffeine, like coffee or chocolate.

❺ Don't take long naps in the day. You can't sleep at night if you sleep too much in the daytime.

---

[10] **tip:** a useful thing to know

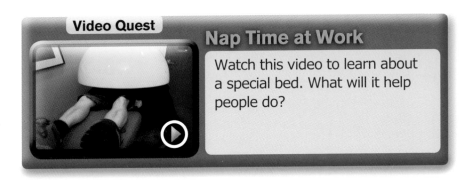

Video Quest

Nap Time at Work

Watch this video to learn about a special bed. What will it help people do?

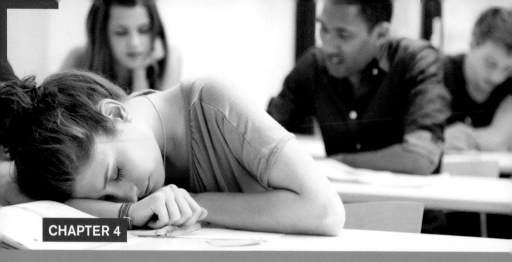

CHAPTER 4

Can't Get Up?

SOME PEOPLE CAN'T SLEEP ENOUGH, BUT OTHER PEOPLE SLEEP TOO MUCH.

Teenagers need more sleep than adults. The brains and bodies of teenagers are growing[11] a lot, so they need more rest. Most high school students need 9 or 10 hours of sleep a day.

Also, teenagers' bodies don't start to get sleepy until 11:00 p.m. or later. And some don't go to bed until 1:00 or 2:00 a.m.! This can be a problem for parents. It's not easy to wake their teenagers up in the morning for school. And when these teenagers get to school, they sometimes **fall asleep** in class.

To help with this problem, some schools in the United States start later in the morning.

[11] **grow:** become bigger and stronger as you get older

Video Quest

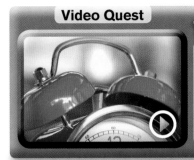

The Get Up and Go!

Watch this video to learn more about the Get Up and Go. How does it wake you up?

It's normal for teenagers to have problems waking up in the morning. But some people can't stay awake at all!

Narcolepsy is a sickness that makes people very sleepy. People with narcolepsy can fall asleep at any time in any place: in a restaurant, at a store, or walking down the street! Narcolepsy can be very dangerous, especially if a narcoleptic person is driving a car.

Another problem is called sleep paralysis. Your mind wakes up, but your body is still asleep. It feels like something heavy is on top of you. You can't move or talk for up to 10 minutes. It's like a nightmare!

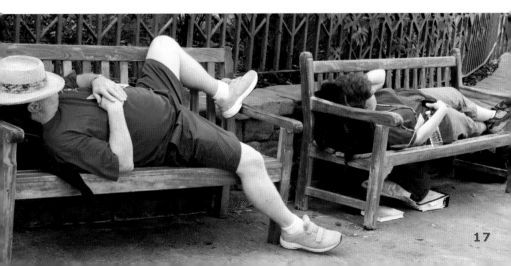

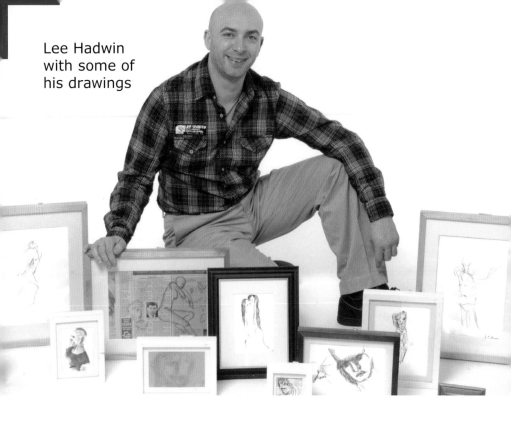

Lee Hadwin
with some of
his drawings

And sometimes people aren't awake, but they walk
and talk and do other things. It's called sleepwalking,
and 30 percent of people in the United States do it at
some time.

Some people do very unusual things when they
sleepwalk. In the day, Lee Hadwin is a nurse.[12]
But when he sleeps at night, he is an artist – he
draws pictures!

When he was a teenager, Lee sleepwalked and drew
pictures on his bedroom walls. Now, he draws beautiful
pictures in all the rooms in his house. He puts paper
and pencils everywhere so he can draw his pictures.

[12] **nurse:** someone who helps people who are sick

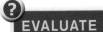

EVALUATE

How are the problems of a narcoleptic and a sleepwalker the same? How are they different?

Some people do very difficult things when they sleepwalk. Robert Wood is a chef, so he cooks in a restaurant in the daytime. But when he sleeps, he cooks, too! Four or five times a week, he sleeps and cooks at the same time.

Most sleepwalkers don't remember doing these things when they wake up. But what about Bizkit, the sleepwalking dog, who runs and barks[13] in his sleep? Does he remember anything when he wakes up?

---

[13] **bark:** A dog doesn't talk, it barks.

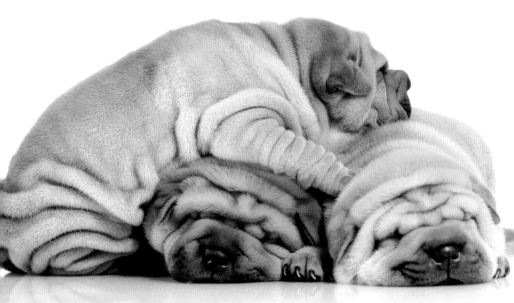

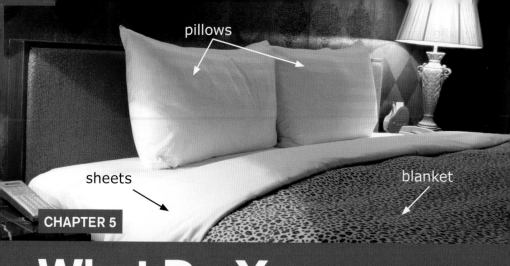

pillows

sheets

blanket

CHAPTER 5

What Do You Think?

A COMFORTABLE BED HELPS PEOPLE GET A GOOD NIGHT'S SLEEP. BUT COMFORTABLE BEDS ARE NOT ALL THE SAME!

What makes a good bed? To start, a **comfortable** mattress and pillows and clean sheets and blankets.

But some people want more than that. They want beds that move. Maybe, they like the cradle bed or the floating bed so they can rock themselves to sleep.

Other people like beds that have a top over part of them. Maybe the top makes them feel safe. These beds are like the egg pod Lady Gaga came out of on the 2011 Grammy Awards TV show. Lady Gaga uses the egg pod as a bed in her New York home.

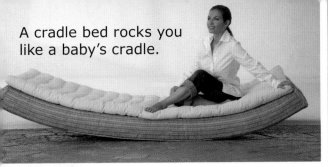

A cradle bed rocks you like a baby's cradle.

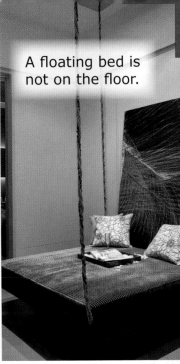

A floating bed is not on the floor.

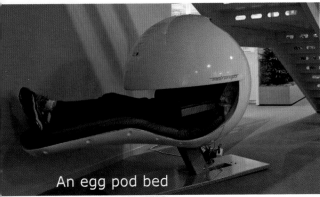

An egg pod bed

And some people like beds that are comfortable but also fun. They sleep in beds that look like hamburgers, cars, guitars, or many other things.

We spend so much time sleeping, it's important to feel comfortable in our beds and enjoy them, too.

Think about your bed. What do you like about it? What don't you like about it? Do you want a bed that moves or has a top or looks like something special?

Video Quest

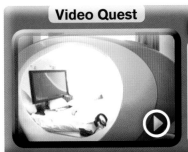

Bedrooms of the Future

Watch this video to learn about the bedrooms of tomorrow. What will be different about bedrooms in the future?

After You Read

Read the sentences and choose Ⓐ (True) or Ⓑ (False).

1 In one year, we spend about four months sleeping.
   Ⓐ True
   Ⓑ False

2 New babies need 14 hours of sleep a day.
   Ⓐ True
   Ⓑ False

3 We dream during REM sleep.
   Ⓐ True
   Ⓑ False

4 Not everyone dreams.
   Ⓐ True
   Ⓑ False

5 Some adults need more sleep than others.
   Ⓐ True
   Ⓑ False

6 It's not good to watch TV right before you go to bed.
   Ⓐ True
   Ⓑ False

Video
7 In America, 16 percent of workers are late for work once a week.
   Ⓐ True
   Ⓑ False

8 Narcolepsy is when you wake up but can't move your body.
   Ⓐ True
   Ⓑ False

Choose the Correct Answers

Circle all of the answers that are correct for each item.

1 During REM sleep _____.

    (A) our eyes move a lot and very fast

    (B) we have dreams or nightmares

    (C) our bodies get the energy they need

2 Dreaming can help you _____.

    (A) repair your body

    (B) remember things

    (C) solve a problem

3 Not enough sleep is bad for your health because _____.

    (A) it can make you sad and depressed

    (B) it can give you headaches

    (C) it can make you eat more

4 Teenagers need more sleep than adults because _____.

    (A) they are busier

    (B) their brains are growing a lot

    (C) their bodies are growing a lot

Complete the Text

Use the words in the box to complete the paragraph.

awake	move	repair	rested	sleep

    Good sleep is important. Our bodies **1** _____
themselves while we sleep. And when we feel **2** _____ ,
we can work and study much better. Many people have trouble sleeping.
Some people have narcolepsy and can't stay **3** _____
during the day. Other people have sleep paralysis. They wake up but can't
4 _____ their bodies. And some people walk, cook, or
even paint pictures while they **5** _____ .

Answer Key

Words to Know, page 4
1 dream **2** nightmare **3** nap **4** relax **5** brain **6** snore

Words to Know, page 5
1 awake **2** rested **3** mind **4** sleepy **5** fall asleep

Analyze, page 7 *Answers will vary.*

Analyze, page 11
Possible answer: We have the same problems or want the same things again and again.

Video Quest, page 15
It helps people to get up in the morning.

Video Quest, page 17
It shakes you.

Evaluate, page 19
Possible answer: The narcoleptic can't control his sleep during the day. The sleepwalker can't control his sleep during the night.

Video Quest, page 21
They will be like very small rooms with everything you need in one place. They don't use much energy and are never too hot or too cold.

True or False?, page 22
1 A **2** B **3** A **4** B **5** A **6** A **7** A **8** B

Choose the Correct Answers, page 23
1 a, b **2** b, c **3** a, b, c **4** b, c

Complete the Text, page 23
1 repair **2** rested **3** awake **4** move **5** sleep